I0413843

Ketogenic Diet: Easy, Fast and Yummy

SUNNY HEBB

Copyright © 2017 Sunny Hebb

TABLE OF CONTENTS

PART 1: INTRODUCTION

I want to thank you and congratulate you for downloading my book "Ketogenic Diet: Easy, Fast and Yummy".

Some people follow the ketogenic diet as a mean of losing weight. Because ketosis breaks down fat that is stored within our bodies, some diets' goal is to create this state of metabolism, so as to aid in losing weight. Ketos diets are also known under the name of LCHF (low carb, high fat) diets. It can be regarded as the diet with lots of fats, with approximately 75% of calories being derived from fat. On the other hand, about 20% of calories are from proteins and 5% from carbohydrates.

Sticking to the ketogenic diet can lead to short term losing weight. A study that was conducted in 2008 revealed that obese men who followed a ketogenic diet for 28 days lost an average of

12 lbs during this period. While following the diet, the participants were able to consume fewer calories without having the urge to eat.

BENEFITS AND DANGERS OF THE KETOGENIC DIET

At first, switching to a ketogenic diet plan may be difficult because the metabolism of one's body is adapting to fat burning rather than depend on glucose. However, it's good to know that most of the symptoms can be avoided. During the first seven days on this diet, the levels of blood sugar will drop, and one may experience an overload of insulin and reactive hypothermia. This usually happens to people who are resistant to insulin.

It takes approximately three days to burn through all the glycogen that is stored in the muscles and liver. A ketogenic diet also has the ability to alter the water and mineral balance in a person's body, so, adding extra salt to the food and taking mineral supplements may be helpful. Try taking sodium, potassium, and magnesium on a daily basis to reduce the side effects.

If you follow a ketogenic diet plan and adapted to it, you will feel much better and healthier. One of the health gains of this diet is that it will lower your fasting blood sugar as well as the levels of insulin. Furthermore, it also aids in the reversal of insulin resistant conditions such as type 2 diabetes, fatty liver, and metabolic syndrome.

In case you have doubts, please remember that there is a lot of credible research that has shown how following a ketogenic diet plan is not harmful to the health of humans. It is only when one consumes too much fat and a lot of carbs that have a negative impact on your health. The sugar that comes from the carbohydrates increases the levels of insulin, and those high levels of insulin interrupt the normal fat metabolism. More fat is stored or circulated in the bloodstream.

This results in the metabolic syndrome and

weight that is linked with resistance to insulin and begins the health issues associated with a diet high in carbohydrates, not a ketogenic diet plan.

LOSING WEIGHT

A ketogenic diet is an effective way of losing weight apart from lowering risks of ailments. Research has revealed that ketogenic diets are far more effective than the recommended low-fat diets. Furthermore, the ketogenic diet is so filling that one can shed weight without counting calories or monitor the food you eat.

Another study also found out that people on a ketogenic diet lost two times more weight than those on a calorie-restricted low-fat diet plan. Their triglyceride, as well as HDL levels, also improved. It was also found out in a separate study that people on a ketogenic diet lost three times more weight than those on diabetes recommended diet.

Several reasons exist as to why a ketogenic diet is better than a low-fat diet.one of them is the increased consumption of protein which offers benefits. In a nutshell, ketogenic diets aid one in losing weight than diets with low fat. All this happens without hunger.

DIABETES AND PREDIABETES

This diet enables you to lose excessive fat, which is closely connected to type 2 diabetes, prediabetes as well as metabolic syndrome. Several studies have been done to prove that this diet aids with diabetes. One of them found out that this diet improved the sensitivity of insulin by a whopping 75%.

Another also investigated people with type 2 diabetes. It found out that seven out of the twenty-one participants were able to stop all medications related to diabetes. All these show that this diet can boost insulin sensitivity and trigger loss of fat, which results in the improvement of type 2 diabetes and prediabetes.

IMPROVING PARKINSON'S SYMPTOMS

Since this diet reduces the levels of insulin, it plays a key role in polycystic ovary syndrome

A study also found out that the ketogenic diet reduces concussions and aids in recovery for those with brain injuries.

For those suffering from acne, lower levels of insulin, as well as consumption of less sugar and processed foods, is beneficial.

SUPRESSING APPETITE

Feeling hungry is the worst side effect of being on a diet. It is one of the major reasons that many people give up on their dieting programs. One of the advantages of eating a low carb diet leads to an automatic appetite reduction.

Studies have shown that when people cut carbs and consume more protein and fat, they end up consuming fewer calories.

FAT LOSS IN THE ABDOMINAL CAVITY

Not all fats in the body are alike. Where fat is stored determines how it affects health as well as the risk of illness.it is important to know that we have fat under the skin and in the abdominal cavity. The fat that tends to be lodged around the organs is what is known as visceral fat. A lot of fat in such areas can trigger inflammation, resistance to insulin and is responsible for metabolism syndrome. Diets low in carbs are quite effective in the reduction of such abdominal fat that is harmful.

REDUCTION OF TRIGLYCERIDES

Triglycerides are molecules of fat. Consumption of carbs drives up levels of triglycerides, especially sugar. When a person cuts down on carbs, they experience a reduction in blood triglycerides.

INCREASING OF GOOD CHOLESTEROL

The higher the levels of HDL, the lower the risk of heart ailments. One of the best ways to raise levels of HDL is to consume fat and diets low in carb.

LDL is bad cholesterol and is linked to heart attacks. A diet that is low on carbs transform LDL particles from small to large, and at the same time reducing the number of LDL particles that float in the bloodstream.

REDUCTION OF BLOOD SUGAR AND INSULIN

When we consume carbohydrates, they are broken down into glucose in the digestive tract. After that, they enter the bloodstream and raise the levels of blood sugar. Since high levels of blood sugar are toxic, the body responds through insulin. For healthy people, the rapid response of insulin minimizes the blood sugar surge in order to prevent it from being harmful to us.

However, many people have the resistance of insulin. This means that the cells do not detect the insulin making it difficult for the body to take blood sugar into the cells. This can lead to type 2 diabetes. By reducing intake of carbs, you eliminate the need for insulin. Both the blood sugar and insulin levels decrease.

REDUCTION OF BLOOD PRESSURE

Low carb diets are effective in the reduction of blood pressure, and this reduces the risk of diseases.

OTHER HEALTH BENEFITS

The ketogenic diet initially came about as a tool for the treatment of neurological disorders like epilepsy. It also can improve body fat, HDL levels, blood pressure and blood sugar. Furthermore, this diet is also being used in the treatment of several cancer types and slowing of tumor growths. It also reduces the symptoms of Alzheimer's and slows down its progress. In epilepsy, it reduces seizures.

Ketogenic diet is the most effective in the treatment of metabolic syndrome. The symptoms are: abdominal obesity, increased blood pressure, increased fasting blood sugar levels, high triglycerides, low HDL levels. All these symptoms improve on a low carb diet.

PART 2: TWO-WEEK MEAL PLAN WITH SHOPPING LISTS

FIRST WEEK MEAL PLAN

MONDAY

Breakfast: Keto Pizza Waffles

Lunch: Southern Pork Stew

Dinner: Herbed Salmon with Roasted Mushrooms

Smoothies: Ginger Grapefruit Green Smoothie

Per Day:

Calories: 1840; Fat: 152g; Protein: 79g; Carbs: 39g; Fiber: 14g; Net Carbs: 25g.

Fat 74% • Protein 20% • Carbs 6%

TUESDAY

Breakfast: Morning Muffins

Lunch: Keto Bacon Chicken Sandwich with Avocado

Dinner: Layered Taco Bake

Smoothies: Tropical Kiwi Smoothie

Per Day:

Calories: 1725; Fat: 139g; Protein: 87g; Carbs: 26g; Fiber: 10g; Net Carbs: 16g.

Fat 74% • Protein 21% • Carbs 5%

WEDNESDAY

Breakfast: Keto Waffles with Pumpkin Spice

Lunch: Spring Salad

Dinner: Pizza Lasagna

Smoothies: Veggie-Packed Green Smoothie

Per Day:

Calories: 1607; Fat: 123g; Protein: 77g; Carbs: 34g; Fiber: 17g; Net Carbs: 17g.

Fat 77% • Protein 19% • Carbs 4%

THURSDAY

Breakfast: Keto Cheese Tacos

Lunch: Chicken Egg Soup

Dinner: Baked Coconut Shrimp

Smoothies: Cucumber Lemonade

Per Day:

Calories: 1637; Fat: 137g; Protein: 79g; Carbs: 26g; Fiber: 6g; Net Carbs: 20g.

Fat 75% • Protein 20% • Carbs 5%

FRIDAY

Breakfast: Keto Donuts

Lunch: Jalapeno Mug Cake

Dinner: Baked Chicken with Zucchini

Smoothies: Tropical Raspberry Smoothie

Per Day:

Calories: 1635; Fat: 134g; Protein: 85g; Carbs: 21g; Fiber: 7g; Net Carbs: 14g.

Fat 74% • Protein 21% • Carbs 5%

SATURDAY

Breakfast: Chive and Bacon Omelet

Lunch: Enchilada Soup

Dinner: Provolone and Prosciutto Stuffed Meatloaf

Smoothies: Raspberry Almond Smoothie

Per Day:

Calories: 1633; Fat: 137g; Protein: 81g; Carbs: 19g; Fiber: 5g; Net Carbs: 14g.

Fat 76% • Protein 20% • Carbs 4%

SUNDAY

Breakfast: Brie and Raspberry Stuffed Waffles

Lunch: Keto Peper and Basil Pizza

Dinner: Smothered Chicken

Smoothies: Avocado Fat Burning Smoothie

Per Day:

Calories: 1712; Fat: 143g; Protein: 79g; Carbs: 27g; Fiber: 13g; Net Carbs: 14g.

Fat 74% • Protein 21% • Carbs 5%

FIRST WEEK SHOPPING LIST

MEAT AND SEAFOOD

Bacon (44 slices)

Chicken breast, 1 boneless (6 ounces)

Chicken, ground (1 pound)

Salmon, smoked (2 ounces)

DAIRY, DAIRY ALTERNATIVES, AND EGGS

Almond milk (2 cups)

Butter (2 cups)

Coconut cream (¾ cup)

Coconut milk beverage (3 cups)

Cream cheese (5 ounces)

Eggs (20)

Goat cheese (12 ounces)

PRODUCE

Avocados (4)

Blueberries (1 pint)

Cauliflower (2)

Celeriac (1)

English cucumber (1)

Lemons (2)

Mint sprigs, fresh (1 bunch)

Onion, sweet (1)

Oregano, fresh (1 bunch)

Raspberries (1 pint)

Tomato (2)

Zucchini (4)

CANNED AND BOTTLED ITEMS

Almond butter (2 cups)

Coconut milk (2 cups)

Coconut oil (2 cups)

Olive oil (1 cup)

Olive oil, extra-virgin (2 tablespoons)

Vanilla extract, alcohol-free (2 teaspoons)

PANTRY ITEMS

Almonds, ground (1¾ cup)

Almonds, sliced (1 cup)

Coconut, shredded unsweetened (4 cups)

Peanut butter (2 tablespoons)

Pine nuts (¼ cup)

Protein powder, chocolate (2 tablespoons)

Protein powder, plain (4 tablespoons)

Protein powder, vanilla (8 tablespoons)

Vanilla bean (2)

Walnuts, chopped (10 ounces)

SECOND WEEK MEAL PLAN

MONDAY

Breakfast: Baked Avocado with Eggs and Bacon

Lunch: Breezy Caprese Salad

Dinner: Lemon and Garlic Roasted Chicken

Smoothies: Gingered Plum Smoothie

Per Day:

Calories: 1622; Fat: 126g; Protein: 88g; Carbs: 34g; Fiber: 15g; Net Carbs: 19g.

Fat 70% • Protein 22% • Carbs 8%

TUESDAY

Breakfast: Super Green Smoothie

Lunch: Keto Peanut Shrimp Curry

Dinner: Tex-Mex Chicken Casserole

Smoothies: Nutty Fat Bomb Smoothie

Per Day:

Calories: 1606; Fat: 130g; Protein: 77g; Carbs: 35g; Fiber: 17g; Net Carbs: 18g.

Fat 73% • Protein 20% • Carbs 7%

WEDNESDAY

Breakfast: Lavender Biscuits

Lunch: Cucumber Salad

Dinner: Stuffed Bacon Cheeseburgers

Smoothies: Cinnamon Roll Smoothie

Per Day:

Calories: 1604; Fat: 130g; Protein: 86g; Carbs: 23g; Fiber: 9g; Net Carbs: 14g.

Fat 73% • Protein 21% • Carbs 6%

THURSDAY

Breakfast: Peachy Chia Jam

Lunch: Pizzas on Portobello

Dinner: Broccoli Beef Bake

Smoothies: Minty Keto Milkshake

Per Day:

Calories: 1720; Fat: 140g; Protein: 83g; Carbs: 32g; Fiber: 13g; Net Carbs: 19g.

Fat 73% • Protein 20% • Carbs 7%

FRIDAY

Breakfast: Keto Style McMuffin

Lunch: Gingere Glazed Salmon

Dinner: Deep Dish Pizza

Smoothies: Pineapple Green Smoothie

Per Day:

Calories: 1707; Fat: 139g; Protein: 84g; Carbs: 30g; Fiber: 7g; Net Carbs: 23g.

Fat 73% • Protein 20% • Carbs 7%

SATURDAY

Breakfast: Goat Cheese and Spinach Omelet

Lunch: Egg Stuffed Avocado

Dinner: Stuffed Cabbage Enchiladas

Smoothies: Chocolate Peanut Butter Shake

Per Day:

Calories: 1651; Fat: 142g; Protein: 75g; Carbs: 20g; Fiber: 5g; Net Carbs: 14g.

Fat 76% • Protein 20% • Carbs 4%

SUNDAY

Breakfast: Creamy Coconut Yogurt

Lunch: Keto tomato Pesto Mug Cake

Dinner: Hoisin-Soy Pork Tenderloin

Smoothies: Strawberry Cheesecake Smoothie

Per Day:

Calories: 1697; Fat: 140g; Protein: 71g; Carbs: 31g; Fiber: 13g; Net Carbs: 18g.

Fat 74% • Protein 20% • Carbs 6%

SECOND WEEK SHOPPING LIST

MEAT AND SEAFOOD

Bacon (14 slices)

Chicken breast, 2 boneless (6 ounces each)

Chicken thighs, bone-in, skin on (4)

Haddock fillets, 4 boneless (5 ounces each)

Sausage, preservative-free or homemade (1 pound)

Sea scallops (1 pound)

Turkey, ground (1½ pounds)

DAIRY, DAIRY ALTERNATIVES, AND EGGS

Almond milk (2 cups)

Butter (1¼ cups)

Coconut cream (¾ cup)

Coconut milk beverage (½ cup)

Cream cheese (1¾ cups)

Eggs (20)

PRODUCE

Avocados (4)

Button mushrooms (1 pound)

Cauliflower (2)

Cilantro (1 bunch)

Kale (1 bunch)

Lemons (3)

Onions, sweet (2)

Oregano, fresh (1 bunch)

Raspberries (2 pints)

Tomato (1)

Zucchini (4)

CANNED AND BOTTLED ITEMS

Almond butter (2 cups)

Chicken stock (4¾ cups)

Coconut oil (1¾ cups)

Olive oil (½ cup)

Olive oil, extra-virgin (6 tablespoons)

Vanilla extract, alcohol-free (2 teaspoons)

PANTRY ITEMS

Almond flour (1½ cups)

Almonds, sliced (1 cup)

Baking powder (½ teaspoon)

Cocoa powder (¼ cup)

Coconut, shredded unsweetened (3¼ cups)

Nutritional yeast (2 teaspoons)

Onion powder (½ teaspoon)

Peanut butter (6 tablespoons)

Protein powder, chocolate (2 tablespoons)

Protein powder, plain (2 tablespoons)

Protein powder, vanilla (2 tablespoons)

PART 3: KETOGENIC RECIPES

BREAKFAST RECIPES

Keto Pizza Waffles

This recipe will produce 2 waffles.

Ingredients:

- 1 tablespoon butter (or bacon grease)
- 1 teaspoon baking powder
- 3 tablespoons almond flour
- 1 teaspoon Italian seasoning
- 1 tablespoon psyllium husk powder
- 4 tablespoons Parmesan cheese
- 3 oz cheddar cheese
- 4 large eggs
- ½ cup tomato sauce
- 14 pepperoni slices (If you're aiming for a classic pizza)
- salt and pepper to taste

Preparation:

1. Add everything except your sauce, cheeses and toppings to an immersion blender and mix together until thick and free of clumps.

2. Heat your waffle iron and add half your blended mixture. Many waffle irons have a handy little light that will tell you when it's ready but if not, look for the flow of steam coming from the iron to almost disappear to indicate it is ready.

3. Repeat step 2 with the rest of your mixture.

4. Add half your tomato sauce (¼ cup) and half your cheese (1.5 oz.) to each pizza waffle.

5. Add your pepperoni, or any other toppings, to the pizzas.

6. Broil for a few minutes until the cheese begins to bubble and crisp. For cheddar, broiling generally takes about 3-5 minutes, but this time will vary with other cheeses so keep

an eye on it!

And there you go, two delicious pizza waffles for breakfast!

Per serving:

Calories: 525: Fat: 41g: Protein: 29 g; Carbs: 5g.

Morning Muffins

This recipe yields 6 muffins.

Ingredients:

- 1 teaspoon vanilla extract
- 2 tablespoons coconut oil
- ½ teaspoon salt
- ½ teaspoon baking powder
- 1 tablespoon cinnamon
- ¼ cup cocoa power
- 1 teaspoon apple cider vinegar
- ¼ cup slivered almonds
- ½ cup pumpkin puree
- 1 large egg
- 1 cup golden flaxseed meal
- ¼ cup sugar-free caramel syrup

Preparation:

1. Set your oven to 350° F.

2. Combine all your wet ingredients in one bowl and mix well. Do the same to your dry

ingredients in a separate bowl.

3. Now pour your wet ingredients into the dry and mix. Pour slowly and be sure to mix well in order to prevent clumping.

4. Set 6 standard paper liners into your muffin tin and add roughly ¼ cup of your mixture to each liner.

5. Sprinkle the almond slivers over the tops of the muffins for a little garnish and crunch (a dramatic flair while sprinkling is optional).

6. Bake the muffins for 15 minutes and check. Once the muffins rise and are set then you'll know they're ready.

Quick, easy and your sweet tooth will thank you.

Per serving:

Calories: 185 g; Fat: 13g; Protein: 7.5g; Carbs: 3.5g.

Keto Waffles with Pumpkin Spice

This recipe yields 2 servings.

Ingredients:

- 1 teaspoon baking powder
- 1 teaspoon vanilla extract
- 3 tablespoons Swerve sweetener
- 1½ teaspoons pumpkin pie spice
- 1/3 cup coconut milk
- ½ cup almond flour
- 2 tablespoons flaxseed meal
- ¼ cup canned pumpkin
- 2 large eggs
- 7 drops liquid stevia

Preparation:

1. Mix all your wet ingredients in a large bowl. Be sure to mix well until no egg whites are visible.

2. Combine all dry ingredients in a sifter.

3. Sift all dry ingredients into the wet

ingredients and mix as you go. If you don't have a sifter, simply mixing all the dry ingredients in a bowl and slowly sprinkling them into the wet ingredients will work too.

4. Mix the wet and dry ingredients until they are fully combined. Your mixture will be a little watery, but don't worry!

5. Heat and grease your waffle iron. Coconut spray gives your waffles a fantastic hint of coconut!

6. Pour your mixture into the iron and cook until the built-in alarm goes off, or the stream of steam begins to dissipate. Serve 'em up with your favorite syrup or fruit!

Per serving:

Calories: 290; Fat: 25g; Protein: 14g; Carbs: 2g.

Keto Cheese Tacos

This recipe yields 3 servings.

Ingredients:

- 3 strips bacon
- 1 oz cheddar cheese (shredded)
- ½ avocado
- 2 tablespoons butter
- 1 cup mozzarella cheese (shredded)
- 6 large eggs
- salt and pepper to taste

Preparation:

1. Start by fully cooking the bacon. Either in an oven for 15 to 20 minutes at 375° F or stovetop.

2. Heat a clean pan over medium heat and add 1/3 cup of mozzarella.

3. Heat the cheese until it just begins to bubble and turn brown on the side touching the pan. Pay close attention here! It will only take a few

seconds for the cheese to jump from brown to burned.

4. Slip a spatula under the cheese and gently unstick it from the pan.

5. Now use a pair of tongs and drape the cheese over a wooden spoon, which should be resting over a bowl or pot. Allow the cheese to cool and form a taco shell shape.

6. Repeat steps 2 to 5 with the rest of your mozzarella.

7. Now add your butter and eggs to the pan and cook completely, adding salt and pepper to suit your taste.

8. Divide the eggs equally between your cheese shells.

9. Slice the avocado and divide the slices evenly between the tacos.

10. Chop or crumble your bacon and again divide equally between the tacos.

11. Last step! Sprinkle your cheddar cheese over the tops. All done!

Per serving:

Calories: 445; Fat: 36g; Protein: 26g; Carbs: 4g.

Keto Donuts

This recipe yields 22 servings (one donut per serving).

Ingredients:

- 4 tablespoons almond flour
- 1 tablespoon coconut flour
- 1 teaspoon vanilla extract
- 1 teaspoon baking powder
- 4 tablespoon erythritol
- 3 oz cream cheese
- 3 large eggs
- 10 drops liquid stevia

Preparation:

1. Add all of your ingredients to a bowl or pitcher and combine with an immersion blender. A food processor will also work for this step if you don't have an immersion blender.

2. Make sure that all your ingredients are well blended and smooth.

3. Heat your donut maker and spray with your grease of choice. Coconut oil always gives your cooking a savory finish!

4. Pour your mixture into the donut maker. Don't fill all the way to the top, leave some room (say 10%) to give your donuts space to rise.

5. Let the mixture cook for 3 minutes and then flip and cook a further 2 minutes.

6. Remove the cooked donuts and repeat steps 3 to 5 for the rest of your batter.

Voilà! You've just created 22 delicious keto friendly donuts.

Per serving:

Calories: 30; Fat: 2.5g; Protein: 1.5g; Carbs: 0.5g.

Chive and Bacon Omelet

This recipe yields 1 serving.

Ingredients:

- 1 oz cheddar cheese
- 1 teaspoon bacon fat
- 2 slices bacon (cooked)
- 2 stalks cheddar
- 2 large eggs
- salt and pepper to taste

Preparation:

1. Make sure your chives are chopped, cheese shredded, eggs are cracked and mixed and bacon cooked before you begin. Omelet making tends to be a fast process so keep on your toes and don't waste time completing these steps later!

2. Heat your bacon fat in a pan on medium-low heat.

3. Add your eggs, chives and salt and pepper

to the pan.

4. Cook until you can see the edges start to set and then cook for another 30 seconds.

5. Immediately add your bacon to the center of the omelet and turn off the heat.

6. Sprinkle your cheese on top of the bacon.

7. Fold two edges of the egg on top of the bacon/cheese pile. The melted cheese should hold the egg in place.

8. Repeat step 7 with the rest of the egg. This will create a slightly burrito shaped omelet.

9. Flip the omelet over and allow it to cook a little longer in the pan (it'll still be warm).

10. Feel free to sprinkle some extra chive, cheese, or bacon on top.

A very fast paced recipe, but it'll leave you with a delicious start to the day.

Per serving:

Calories: 460; Fat: 36g; Protein: 25g; Carbs: 2g.

Brie and Raspberry Stuffed Waffles

This recipe yields 2 servings.

Ingredients:

Waffles

- 1 teaspoon vanilla extract
- 1 teaspoon baking powder
- 2 tablespoons flaxseed meal
- ½ cup almond flour
- 2 tablespoons Swerve sweetener
- 7 drops liquid stevia
- 2 large eggs
- 1/3 cup coconut milk

Filling

- 1 tablespoon lemon juice
- 1 tablespoon Swerve sweetener
- ½ cup raspberries
- zest of ½ lemon
- 2 tablespoons butter
- 3 oz cream brie

Preparation:

1. Mix all the waffle ingredients in a container. Make sure your batter is smooth with no lumps.

2. Heat your waffle maker and once it's hot, add your mixture.

3. Cook until either the indicator light says its ready or the steam dissipates.

4. Remove your waffles and repeat as necessary to cook all of your batters.

5. Slice your brie and drape over two of your four waffles. The waffles will still be warm and this will melt the brie.

6. In a pan, heat the Swerve sweetener and butter

7. Just as the butter begins to bubble; add your raspberries, lemon juice and zest.

8. Stir your raspberry mixture until it just begins to bubble. As the mixture lets off steam, it will develop a jam-like consistency and this is

exactly what you want!

9. Now take the two waffle pieces with the brie and broil them until the brie begins to bubble.

10. Pour/spread your raspberry jam on top of the brie waffles and cover with the other two waffles.

11. Grill the assembled waffle sandwich in the pan for a couple minutes until brown and crispy.

Per serving:

Calories: 490; Fat: 40g; Protein: 22g; Carbs: 6g.

Baked Avocados with Eggs and Bacon

This recipe yields 1 serving.

Ingredients:

- 2 small eggs
- 2 slices of bacon
- 1 avocado
- Pepper to taste

Preparation:

1. Pan fry your bacon until it is just barely cooked

2. Preheat your oven to 425° F.

3. Halve the avocado and remove the seed.

4. Crumple some aluminum foil into ring shapes that will hold your avocado halves up on the baking sheet.

5. Break your eggs into a bowl and spoon one yolk into each avocado half. Then continue to fill the hole of each avocado with egg whites

until they're both full.

6. Crumble your bacon and spread on top of the avocados.

7. Add pepper on top and bake in the preheated oven for 12 to 15 minutes. After 10 minutes, check your eggs every minute or two to ensure you don't overcook them!

Serve them up!

Per serving:

Calories: 700; Fat: 60g; Protein: 23g; Carbs: 6g.

Super Green Smoothie

This recipe yields 1 serving.

Ingredients:

- 1 cup baby spinach

- 1 small banana, frozen

- 1 cup unsweetened almond milk

- 1 tablespoon almond butter

- 1 tablespoon coconut oil

- 1 teaspoon sugar-free sweetener

- 5 ice cubes

Preparation:

1. Place all ingredients into your blender and blend on high for 30-60 seconds, until smooth and creamy.

2. If the mixture is too thick, add a bit more almond milk and blend to desired consistency.

3. Serve.

Per serving:

Calories: 311; Fat: 26g; Protein: 6g; Carbs: 17g; Fiber: 4g; Net Carbs: 13g.

Lavender Biscuits

The recipe yields 6 servings.

Ingredients:

- 4 eggs whites
- 1/3 cup coconut oil
- 1½ cups almond flour
- 1 tablespoon lavender buds (culinary grade)
- 1 teaspoon baking powder
- 4 drops liquid stevia
- 1 pinch kosher salt

Preparation:

1. Combine the coconut oil and almond flour in a bowl. Your hands would be the best tool for this job and mix until there are pea-sized clumps of fat throughout the mixture.

2. Put the bowl of flour and oil in the refrigerator.

3. Whip your egg whites until they begin to

foam and add the salt, lavender and baking powder. Mix well.

4. Add the egg mixture to the almond flour and oil and mix well.

5. Use a tablespoon or ice cream scoop to place clumps of the mixture on a greased baking sheet.

6. Give each mound a slight pat so they're not round (think puffy pancake).

7. Bake at 350° F for 20 minutes or until golden brown.

Per serving:

Calories: 270; Fat: 25g; Protein: 10g; Carbs: 4g.

Peachy Chia Jam

This recipe yields 10 servings.

Ingredients:

- 2 tablespoons Swerve sweetener
- 2 tablespoons chia seeds
- 1 teaspoon lemon juice
- 2 cups peaches (chopped)

Preparation:

1. Combine your peaches, lemon juice and sweetener in a blender; and blend until completely smooth.

2. Pour the smooth mixture into a bowl and add your chia seeds. Stir by hand until completely incorporated.

3. Pour your jam mixture into a jar or covered bowl and place in the refrigerator. Let it cool and thicken for about an hour.

All done! Quick recipe and this jam will be the

perfect accompaniment for many of your favorite breakfast pastries!

Per serving:

Calories: 30; Fat: 1g; Protein: 1g; Carbs: 3g.

Keto Style McMuffin

The recipe yields 2 servings.

Ingredients:

Muffins

- 1 large egg
- 2 tablespoons heavy whipping cream
- ¼ teaspoon baking soda
- 2 tablespoons water
- ¼ cup cheddar cheese (grated)
- ¼ cup flax meal
- ¼ cup almond flour
- 1 pinch salt

Filling

- 2 slices cheddar cheese
- 1 tablespoon butter
- 1 tablespoon ghee
- 2 large eggs
- 1 teaspoon Dijon mustard
- 4 slices crisp bacon

- salt and pepper to taste

Preparation:

1. Add all your dry ingredients for the muffins in a large bowl and mix well.

2. Drop in the eggs, cream and water. Mix until completely smooth.

3. Add the grated cheese to the mixture and stir again. Don't worry if the cheese makes it clumpy when you heat it everything will combine nicely.

4. Add your mixture to two single serving ramekins and microwave on high for 60 to 90 seconds.

5. For the filling, cook your eggs on top of the ghee. Don't worry if they're not perfect circles. Do your best and you can trim later.

6. Now cut the cooked muffins in half, and spread your butter on each half.

7. Now stack 'em up! Layer your egg, mustard,

bacon and cheese for each muffin.

All the deliciousness of the classic McMuffin but completely guilt free!

Per serving:

Calories: 315; Fat: 55g; Protein: 26g; Carbs: 3g.

Goat Cheese and Spinach Omelet

The recipe yields 1 serving.

Ingredients:

- 3 large eggs
- 1 medium spring onion
- 1 large handful of spinach
- 2 tablespoons heavy cream
- 2 tablespoons butter
- ¼ onion
- 1 oz goat cheese
- salt and pepper to taste

Preparation:

1. Heat a pan on medium and add the butter. Spread the butter around the pan until it is completely melted.

2. Slice your onion (or dice it) and add to the pan once the butter begins to brown.

3. Caramelize your onion in the butter.

4. Once the onion is fully cooked and caramelized, add your spinach to the pan. Cook until the spinach is wilted.

5. Add salt and pepper to taste, give a final stir and remove the spinach onion mix from the pan and set aside.

6. Now crack your eggs in a container (not the pan!) and add the cream and some salt and pepper. Mix everything together.

7. Now you can add your egg mixture to the pan and cook until the edges just begin to set.

8. Add your onion spinach mixture on one side of the egg, covering about half of the eggs.

9. Crumble your goat cheese over the onion and spinach.

10. Fold the other half of the egg over the top of the onions, spinach and cheese.

11. Remove from pan and garnish with more cheese if you like (who doesn't like more

cheese?).

Per serving:

Calories: 615; Fat: 58g; Protein: 26g; Carbs: 5.4g.

Creamy Coconut Yogurt

The recipe yields 1 serving.

Ingredients:

- 2/3 cup heavy whipping cream
- 2 capsules probiotic-10
- ½ teaspoon xanthan gum
- 1 can coconut milk (full fat)
- toppings (your choice!)

Preparation:

1. Pour the contents of your can of coconut milk into a container and stir well as the water and cream tend to separate (you can do this directly in the can too).

2. Put your coconut milk in a sealable container, and break the probiotic capsules into the milk, mix well, seal the container and place in the oven (with the heat off and the oven light on). Let sit for 12 to 24 hours for the bacteria to culture.

3. After the sitting time, add your yogurt to a bowl and sprinkle in your xanthan gum. Mix completely.

4. In a separate bowl, use an electric mixer to whip your heavy cream until stiff peaks form.

5. Add the cream to the yogurt and mix until you get the consistency you want. You can mix by hand or use an electric mixer if you wish.

6. Add whatever toppings you wish. Any kind of berry is sure to be delicious!

Enjoy your own, homemade, yogurt!

Per serving:

Calories: 310; Fat: 31g; Protein: 0.5g; Carbs: 4.5g.

LUNCH RECIPES

Southern Pork Stew

The recipe yields 4 servings.

Ingredients:

Spices

- 1 teaspoon oregano
- 1 teaspoon paprika
- ¼ teaspoon. cinnamon
- 1 teaspoon minced garlic
- 2 teaspoons cumin
- 2 teaspoons chili powder
- 2 bay leaves
- salt and pepper to taste (approx. ½ teaspoon each)

Meat

1 lb cooked pork shoulder (sliced)

Vegetables

- ½ green bell pepper (sliced)
- ½ red bell pepper (Sliced)
- ½ medium onion
- 6 oz button mushrooms
- ½ jalapeno (sliced)

Soup

- ¼ cup tomato paste
- 2 cups chicken broth
- 2 cups gelatinous bone broth
- Juice: ½ lime
- ½ cup coffee (your remedy for the midday slump)

Preparation:

1. Clean and slice all your vegetables.

2. Add two tablespoons of Olive Oil to a pan and turn to high heat.

3. Sauté your vegetables until they are just beginning to cook and filling your kitchen with

their fantastic aroma. Be careful not to overcook them here! That will give you a slightly mushy stew later on.

4. Set your slow cooker on low; add the bone broth, coffee, and chicken broth.

5. While your slow cooker is warming, add spices and bay leaves to a single bowl. This is a handy step for almost any recipe and will help you keep all your spices in one place.

6. Now add all your mushrooms and sliced pork to the slow cooker.

7. Give your cooking vegetables and oil a final stir and add them to the crock pot along with all your spices.

8. Cover and let the slow cooker work its magic for about 4-10 hours.

9. Once it's finished, remove the bay leaves (or keep an eye out for them) and serve!

A simple, hearty and unique dish to add a little

sunshine to your lunchtime!

Per serving:

Calories: 386; Fat: 29g; Carbs: 6.5g, Protein: 19.8g.

Keto Bacon Chicken Sandwich with Avocado

The recipe yields 2 servings.

Ingredients:

Bread

- ¼ teaspoon salt
- ½ teaspoon garlic powder
- 1/8 teaspoon cream of tartar
- 3 large eggs
- 3 oz cream cheese

Filling

- 3 oz chicken
- 2 slices bacon
- 2 slices pepper jack cheese
- 1 teaspoon sriracha
- 1 tablespoon mayonnaise
- 2 grape tomatoes
- ¼ avocado

Preparation:

1. Preheat oven to 300° F.

2. Separate your eggs into different bowls.

3. Add cream of tartar and salt to the eggs whites and whip until you get soft peaks.

4. Add cream cheese to the egg yolks bowl and beat until a uniform pale yellow color forms.

5. Fold the egg white mixture into the yolks. Gently complete this as we want to keep the whites nice and airy.

6. Line a baking sheet with parchment paper and pour about ¼ cup of your bread mixture into individual areas and form into square shapes.

7. Sprinkle garlic atop the bread and bake for 25 minutes.

8. While the bread is baking, cook the chicken and bacon with a little salt and pepper.

9. Once everything is cooked, assemble your

sandwich with the mayo, avocado, cheese and tomatoes.

Per serving:

Calories: 355; Fat: 28g; Carbs: 1.5g; Protein: 24g.

Spring Salad

This recipe yields 1 serving.

Ingredients:

- 2 tablespoons Parmesan (shaved)
- 2 tablespoons raspberry vinaigrette
- 2 oz mixed greens
- 3 tablespoons pine nuts (roasted)
- 2 slices bacon
- salt and pepper to taste

Preparation:

1. Cook the bacon in a stovetop pan. Nice and crispy is what we're aiming for here!

2. Assemble your salad with the rest of the ingredients and crumble the bacon atop.

3. Shake well to make sure everything in combined

Per serving:

Calories: 470; Fat: 36g; Carbs: 4g; Protein:

17.5g.

Chicken Egg Soup

This recipe yields 1 serving.

Ingredients:

- 2 large eggs
- 1 tablespoon bacon fat
- 1 teaspoon chili garlic paste
- ½ cube chicken bouillon
- 1½ cups chicken broth

Preparation:

1. Heat a pan on medium-high and add the broth, bacon fat and bouillon cube.

2. Once the soup begins to boil, add the chili paste and stir continually for a minute. Now remove from heat.

3. Beat the eggs in a separate container and pour into the broth.

4. Stir and let sit for about 30 seconds.

Per serving:

Calories: 275; Fat: 24g; Carbs: 2g; Protein: 13g.

Jalapeno Mug Cake

This recipe yields 1 serving.

Ingredients:

- 1 large egg
- 1 tablespoon cream cheese
- 1 tablespoon butter
- 1 slice bacon
- ½ teaspoon baking powder
- ½ jalapeno pepper
- 2 tablespoons almond flour
- 1 tablespoon golden flaxseed meal
- ¼ teaspoon salt

Preparation:

1. Heat a pan over medium and cook the bacon until nice and crisp.

2. Now in a mug, mix all of the remaining ingredients. Scrape down the sides so everything is in the bottom of the mug.

3. Microwave for 80 seconds on high.

4. Flip the mug upside down and gently tap against a plate to make the cake fall out, and garnish with the bacon and any leftover jalapenos.

Per serving:

Calories: 430; Fat: 36g; Carbs: 5g; Protein: 16g.

Enchilada Soup

The recipe yields 4 servings.

Ingredients:

- 8 oz cream cheese
- 4 cups chicken broth
- 6 oz chicken (shredded)
- 4 stalks celery (diced)
- 1 red bell pepper (diced)
- 3 tablespoons olive oil
- ½ teaspoon cayenne pepper
- ½ lime (juiced)
- 2 teaspoons cumin
- 1 teaspoon chili powder
- 1 teaspoon oregano
- 2 teaspoons garlic
- 1 cup tomatoes (diced)
- ½ cup cilantro (chopped)

Preparation:

1. Heat the olive oil in a pan on medium. Once hot, add the celery and pepper.

2. Once the celery is soft, toss in your tomatoes and cook until they begin to release their juice.

3. Add all your spices to the pan and stir several times to incorporate.

4. Now add your cilantro and chicken broth to the pot and crank up the heat to bring to a boil.

5. Once boiling, reduce heat to low and simmer for 25 minutes.

6. Now add your cream cheese and again bring to a boil, then reduce heat and simmer again for 30 minutes.

7. Add the shredded chicken to the pot as well as the lime juice. Stir several times to make sure everything is well mixed.

All set! Feel free to garnish with some cilantro or more cheese!

Per serving:

Calories: 350; Fat: 30g; Carbs: 5g; Protein:

14g.

Keto Pepper and Basil Pizza

This recipe yields 2 servings (½ of one pizza).

Ingredients:

Crust

- 1 large egg
- 2 tablespoons cream cheese
- 2 tablespoons psyllium husk
- 1 teaspoon Italian seasoning
- 2 tablespoons Parmesan cheese
- 6 oz mozzarella cheese
- ½ cup almond flour
- ½ tsp. each of salt and pepper

Toppings

- ¼ cup tomato sauce
- 3 tablespoons fresh basil (chopped)
- 4 oz cheddar cheese (shredded)
- 2/3 bell pepper
- 1 vine tomato

Preparation:

1. Preheat your oven to 400° F.

2. Give your mozzarella (for the crust) a quick 45-second zap in the microwave to melt it.

3. Add all the other crust ingredients to the cheese and mix together completely.

4. Use your hands, or a rolling pin, to flatten the dough and make a circle.

5. Bake this for 10 minutes and remove from the oven.

6. Now throw on all your toppings and bake for an additional 10 minutes.

7. Remove pizza and let it cool

Per serving:

Calories: 420; Fat: 30g; Carbs: 6g; Protein: 25g.

Breezy Caprese Salad

This recipe yields 2 servings.

Ingredients:

- 3 tablespoons olive oil
- 6 oz mozzarella cheese
- 1 tomato
- ¼ cup fresh basil (chopped)
- black pepper and salt to taste

Preparation:

1. Use a blender, or food processor, to pulse the basil and olive oil. This will leave you will a basil paste.

2. Now slice your tomato into about ¼-inch slices. We're looking for 6 slices here, so feel free to grab another tomato if you need to!

3. Cut the mozzarella into 1 oz slices (right about the same size as the tomatoes or slightly thicker).

4. Layer your Caprese with the tomato as the base, then cheese and topped with basil paste.

5. Season with salt and pepper to taste.

Feel free to garnish with extra olive oil.

Per serving:

Calories: 406; Fat: 35g; Carbs: 5g; Protein: 17g.

Keto Peanut Shrimp Curry

This recipe yields 2 servings.

Ingredients:

- 1 teaspoon fish sauce
- 1 tablespoon peanut butter
- 1 teaspoon ginger (minced)
- 1 teaspoon roasted garlic (crushed)
- 1 tablespoon soy sauce
- ¼ teaspoon xanthan gum
- ½ teaspoon turmeric
- 3 tablespoons cilantro (chopped)
- 2 tablespoons coconut oil
- 1 spring onion (chopped)
- 1 cup vegetable stock
- ½ cup sour cream
- 1 cup coconut milk
- 5 oz broccoli florets
- 2 tablespoons green curry paste
- 6 oz shrimp (cooked)
- ½ lime (juiced)

Preparation:

1. Heat a pan over medium and add the coconut oil. When hot, toss in the garlic, spring onion and ginger.

2. Stir for a few minutes; and once cooked, add 1 tablespoon of the green curry paste along with your soy sauce, turmeric, peanut butter and fish sauce.

3. Continue to stir and cook for several minutes.

4. Now add the vegetable broth and coconut milk.

5. Add the xanthan gum and mix completely.

6. When you notice the mixture begin to thicken, toss in the broccoli.

7. Continue to stir and add the cilantro.

8. Lastly; add the shrimp and mix everything up. Allow it to cook for a few more minutes to allow the shrimp taste to develop.

Serve with your sour cream on top and enjoy!

Per serving:

Calories: 450; Fat: 32g; Carbs: 8.5g; Protein: 28g.

Cucumber Salad

This recipe yields 1 serving.

Ingredients:

- ¼ teaspoon red pepper flakes
- 1 tablespoon rice vinegar
- 1 tablespoon sesame oil
- 1 teaspoon sesame seeds
- 2 tablespoons olive oil
- 1 spring onion
- 1 packet shirataki noodles
- ¾ large cucumber
- salt and pepper to taste

Preparation:

1. Thoroughly rinse and wash your shirataki noodles, and allow them to dry on a paper towel.

2. Heat a pan over medium-high and add the coconut oil.

3. Once the pan is hot, add your noodles and

fry them for 6 minutes. They should shrink a great deal and any extra liquid will boil off.

4. Remove the noodles from the pan and again set them on a paper towel to dry.

5. Slice the cucumber into whatever size slices you want and arrange over a plate. Now top the cucumber with all the other ingredients (other than the noodles), and set in the fridge for 30 minutes.

6. Remove from the fridge, top with the noodles and serve.

Per serving:

Calories: 415; Fat: 44g; Carbs: 6g; Protein: 2g.

Pizzas on Portobello

This recipe yields 4 servings.

Ingredients:

- 4 oz mozzarella cheese
- 20 slices pepperoni
- 4 large Portobello mushroom caps
- 1 medium tomato
- 6 tablespoons olive oil
- ¼ cup fresh basil (chopped)
- salt and pepper to taste

Preparation:

1. Scrape the insides out from the mushroom caps. You want to just a have a shell here.

2. Coat the tops (not the insides) of the caps with your olive oil and season with salt and pepper.

3. Broil the mushrooms for about 4 minutes, then flip and broil for an additional 3 to 4 minutes.

4. Slice your tomato into thin pieces and place in the scooped out portion of the mushrooms.

5. Top the tomato with the basil

6. Now top the basil with the pepperoni slices and mozzarella cubes.

7. Broil for 3 to 4 minutes or until cheese starts to bubble.

All set to enjoy!

Per serving:

Calories: 320; Fat: 33g; Carbs: 2.5g; Protein: 8g.

Ginger Glazed Salmon

This recipe yields 2 servings.

Ingredients:

- 1 tablespoon red boat fish sauce
- 2 teaspoons garlic (minced)
- 1 tablespoon ketchup (sugar-free)
- 1 teaspoon ginger (minced)
- 1 tablespoon rice vinegar
- 2 tablespoons white wine
- 2 tablespoons soy sauce
- 2 teaspoons sesame oil
- 10 oz salmon fillet

Preparation:

1. Toss all of your ingredients except for the ketchup, white wine, and sesame oil into a container. Let these marinate for about 15 minutes.

2. Heat a pan on high and add the sesame oil.

3. As soon as the oil lets off a little smoke, add

the fish with the skin side down.

4. Allow the fish skin to crisp up and cook, then flip and continue cooking. It generally takes about 3 to 4 minutes per side. After the first flip, add all the marinade ingredients to the pan and let them cook with the fish.

5. When cooked, remove the salmon from the pan. Add the ketchup and white wine to the liquid left in the pan.

6. Let everything simmer for 6 minutes and put inside the dish.

Serve it up with the sauce on the side.

Per serving:

Calories: 375, Fat: 22 g, Carbs: 2 g, Protein: 34 g.

Egg Stuffed Avocado

This recipe yields 6 servings (each half of avocado is one serving).

Ingredients:

- 2 teaspoons brown mustard
- 1 teaspoon hot sauce
- 4 tablespoons mayonnaise
- 2 tablespoons fresh lime juice
- ½ teaspoon cumin
- 1/3 red onion
- 6 large eggs (hard boiled)
- 3 stalks celery
- 3 avocados
- salt and pepper to taste

Preparation:

1. Chop your onion, celery and hard-boiled eggs.

2. In a bowl, combine all of the ingredients except the avocado.

3. Slice each avocado in half lengthwise and remove the pit.

4. Spoon your egg salad mixture into the center of each avocado slice.

Per serving:

Calories: 300; Fat: 27g; Carbs: 4g; Protein: 8g.

Keto Tomato Pesto Mug Cake

The recipe yields 1 serving.

Ingredients:

- 2 tablespoons butter
- 2 tablespoons almond flour
- 1 large egg
- ½ teaspoon baking powder

Pesto

- 1 tablespoon almond flour
- 5 teaspoons sun-dried tomato pesto
- 1 pinch salt

Preparation:

1. Combine all ingredients in a mug (keep some pesto in reserve if you want it as a topping).

2. Microwave the mug on high for 70 to 80 seconds.

3. Lightly tap the mug against a plate and the

cake will fall out.

4. Top with any leftover pesto.

Quick and easy!

Per serving:

Calories: 460; Fat: 45g; Carbs: 4g; Protein: 13g.

DINNER RECIPES

Herbed Salmon with Roasted Mushrooms

This recipe yields 4 servings.

Ingredients:

- 2 lbs salmon, cut into 4 fillets
- ½ cup sesame oil
- ½ cup tamari (gluten-free soy sauce)
- 1 clove garlic, minced
- 1 teaspoon dried oregano
- ½ teaspoon ground ginger
- ½ teaspoon dried rosemary
- ½ teaspoon dried basil
- ¼ teaspoon dried tarragon
- ¼ teaspoon dried thyme
- ½ cup butter
- ½ cup fresh mushrooms, chopped roughly
- ½ cup chopped green onions

Preparation:

1. Whisk together sesame oil, tamari, minced garlic, herbs and spices in a bowl.

2. Place salmon fillets in large freezer bag and pour sesame oil marinade over fish.

3. Allow salmon to marinate in the refrigerator for 1-4 hours.

4. When the fish is almost finished marinating, preheat oven to 350° F.

5. Line a 9 x 13-inch pan with foil and arrange salmon in a single layer.

6. Cover salmon with remaining marinade and bake for 10-15 minutes.

7. While salmon is baking, melt butter in a skillet over medium-high heat.

8. Add all of the mushrooms and one-half of the green onions to the pan. Stirring occasionally, cook for one minute.

9. Remove salmon from the oven and pour butter mixture, including vegetables, over the fillets.

10. Return to oven to bake for an additional 10 minutes.

11. Top with remaining raw green onions and serve.

Per serving:

Calories 353; Fat: 23g; Carbs: 2g; Protein: 32g.

Layered Taco Bake

This recipe yieldы 7 servings.

Ingredients:

- 2¼ lb lean ground beef
- 2 tablespoons chili powder
- ½ teaspoon garlic powder
- ½ teaspoon onion powder
- ½ teaspoon red pepper flakes
- ½ teaspoon dried oregano
- 1 teaspoon paprika
- 3 teaspoons cumin
- 1 teaspoon salt
- 1 teaspoon black pepper
- ¼ cup water
- 15 oz fire roasted tomatoes, juice reserved
- 15 oz black beans, drained and rinsed
- 6 corn tortillas
- 3 cup sharp cheddar cheese, shredded

Preparation:

1. Preheat oven to 350° F. Grease 2 9-inch pie plates generously.

2. In a large skillet, cook ground beef until no longer pink.

3. Drain fat from beef, and return to skillet. Add spices and water to beef and mix thoroughly to combine.

4. Turn heat to low, and allow beef to simmer. Add fire roasted tomatoes and black beans to the skillet, mixing with the beef.

5. Lay 1 tortilla down in each pie plate. Spoon a quarter of the meat mixture onto each tortilla and top generously with cheese. Layer another tortilla, and divide the remaining meat mixture between the two pie plates. Sprinkle on more cheese. Top each plate with another tortilla and the remaining cheese.

6. Bake uncovered for 25-30 minutes.

7. Serve with 1 tablespoon of sour cream.

Per serving:

Calories 832; Fat: 56g; Carbs: 17g; Protein: 62g.

Pizza Lasagna

This recipe yields 2 servings.

Ingredients:

- 6 oz lean ground beef
- 1 teaspoon Italian seasoning
- 8 slices Canadian bacon
- ¼ cup pizza sauce
- 1 cup mozzarella cheese, shredded
- 3 tablespoons Parmesan cheese, freshly grated

Preparation:

1. Preheat oven to 350° F. Grease a 9-inch pie plate thoroughly.

2. In a skillet, cook ground beef over medium heat until no longer pink. Drain excess fat and season beef with Italian seasoning.

3. Arrange 4 slices of Canadian bacon in the bottom of a pie plate. Spread 1/8 cup of pizza sauce onto bacon and top with half the ground

beef and cheeses. Repeat with remaining Canadian bacon, beef and cheeses.

4. Bake for about 10-15 minutes or until cheese is melted and bubbly.

Per serving:

Calories 702; Fat: 41g; Carbs: 10g; Protein: 75g.

Baked Chicken with Zucchini

This recipe yields 4 servings.

Ingredients:

- 4 boneless, skinless chicken breasts
- 2 medium zucchini, quartered and chopped with seeds removed
- 1 large onion, sliced
- 6 cloves garlic, roughly chopped, plus 4 cloves
- 1 lemon, zested and quartered
- 1 cup chicken broth, plus ¾ cup
- 2 tablespoons melted butter, plus 3 tablespoons
- ¾ cup heavy cream
- 1 tablespoon cornstarch
- 1 tablespoon lemon juice

Preparation:

1. Preheat oven to 400° F. Line a large roasting pan with foil and coat with non-stick spray.

2. Arrange chicken, zucchini, onion, 6 chopped cloves of garlic and lemon quarters in the pan. Sprinkle lightly with salt and pepper.

3. In a small bowl, whisk together 1 cup of chicken broth, 3 tablespoons of melted butter and lemon zest. Pour over chicken.

4. Bake for about 40-45 minutes or until chicken is cooked through.

5. While chicken is baking, melt 3 tablespoons of butter over medium-low heat. Add remaining garlic cloves, and cook for about 2 minutes.

6. Add remaining ¾ cup of broth and heavy cream to saucepan, raising heat to medium-high.

7. In a small bowl, combine cornstarch with 2 tablespoons of water. Stream into the broth, stirring constantly. Let simmer for 5 minutes.

8. Remove pan from heat and stir in lemon juice.

9. Pour sauce over chicken and serve.

Per serving:

Calories 468, Fat: 33 g, Carbs: 10 g. Protein: 30g.

Baked Coconut Shrimp

This recipe yields 4 servings.

Ingredients:

- 18 uncooked jumbo shrimp, peeled and deveined
- 1/3 cup coconut flour
- 1 teaspoon salt
- ½ teaspoon cayenne pepper
- 3 eggs
- 1½ cups unsweetened coconut flakes

Preparation:

1. Preheat oven to 450° F. Spray a wire rack with non-stick spray and place on top of a foil-lined baking sheet.

2. Carve a slit down the center line of each shrimp.

3. On a plate, mix together cornstarch, salt and cayenne pepper.

4. In a small bowl, whisk eggs with a fork.

5. Lay coconut flakes on a separate plate.

6. Dip each shrimp in cornstarch mixture, then eggs, then coconut.

7. Place coated shrimp on a wire rack and lightly spray with non-stick spray.

8. Bake shrimp for 15 minutes, or until cooked through.

Per serving:

Calories 457; Fat: 16g; Carbs: 26g; Protein: 34g.

Provolone & Prosciutto Stuffed Meatloaf

This recipe yields 8 servings.

Ingredients:

- 1 tablespoon butter
- 4 cups raw baby spinach, stems removed
- salt and pepper
- 8 oz tomato sauce
- 6 oz tomato paste
- 2 tablespoons apple cider vinegar
- ¼ cup granulated sweetener, like Splenda
- 1 lb lean ground beef
- 1 lb ground pork
- 3 eggs
- ½ cup Parmesan cheese, freshly grated
- ½ red onion, finely chopped
- ½ red bell pepper, finely chopped
- 4 cloves garlic, minced
- 1 teaspoon dried oregano
- 1 teaspoon dried basil
- 1 teaspoon salt

- ½ teaspoon pepper
- ¼ lb prosciutto, thinly sliced
- ¼ lb Provolone cheese, thinly sliced

Preparation:

1. In a skillet over medium heat, melt butter. Add spinach, season lightly with salt and pepper and cook until leaves are wilted.

2. While spinach is sautéing, mix together tomato sauce, tomato paste, apple cider vinegar and Splenda. Set aside.

3. Preheat oven to 350° F. Line a 9 x 5-inch loaf pan with foil.

4. In a large bowl, thoroughly combine ground meat, eggs, Parmesan cheese, onion, bell pepper, garlic and spices.

5. Lay out a large piece of wax paper. Spread meat mixture into 8 x 10-inch rectangle on paper.

6. Arrange prosciutto slices on top, followed by

cooked spinach and Provolone cheese.

7. Roll meat into a loaf, sealing the ends so that the fillings do not fall out.

8. Lay loaf, seam side down, in the pan. Spread tomato mixture on top. Bake for 1 hour 15 minutes, or until internal temperature reaches 165° F.

Per serving:

Calories 516; Fat: 37g; Carbs: 8g; Protein: 37g.

Smothered Chicken

This recipe yields 8 servings.

Ingredients:

- 4 boneless, skinless chicken breasts
- salt and pepper
- ½ cup barbecue sauce
- 8 slices bacon, cooked and crumbled
- 1½ cups Colby-Jack cheese, shredded

Preparation:

1. Preheat oven to 350° F. Line a baking sheet with foil and spray with non-stick spray.

2. Arrange chicken on prepared baking sheet. Season with salt and pepper and smother with barbecue sauce.

3. Bake for 30 minutes, or until juices run clear.

4. Remove chicken from oven. Top with crumbled bacon and cheese.

5. Return to oven for additional 5 minutes to

melt cheese. Alternately, melt cheese under the broiler.

Per serving:

Calories 570, Fat: 34 g, Carbs: 14 g, Protein: 48 g.

Lemon & Garlic Roasted Chicken

This recipe yields 4 servings.

Ingredients:

- 4 skin-on chicken thighs
- 8 garlic cloves
- 2 lemons
- ¼ cup extra virgin olive oil
- 1 teaspoon salt
- 1 teaspoon pepper
- ½ teaspoon dried oregano
- ½ teaspoon dried basil

Preparation:

1. Preheat oven to 350° F. Line a large roasting pan with foil.

2. Peel garlic cloves and slice lemons into quarters.

3. Arrange chicken in roasting pan, with lemon slices and garlic cloves surrounding them.

4. Season chicken with salt, pepper, oregano and basil. Pour olive oil over chicken to evenly coat.

5. Bake for 45-60 minutes or until chicken is cooked through.

Per serving:

Calories 413; Fat: 38g; Carbs: 3g; Protein: 17g.

Tex-Mex Chicken Casserole

This recipe yields 8 servings.

Ingredients:

- 2 tablespoons extra virgin olive oil
- 8 chicken breasts, cubed
- 1 tablespoon chili powder
- 1 teaspoon cumin
- 1 teaspoon garlic powder
- ½ teaspoon onion powder
- ½ teaspoon salt
- ½ teaspoon pepper
- 1 cup sour cream
- 4 oz fire-roasted green chilies
- 16 oz jarred salsa
- 1 cup Monterey cheese, shredded
- 1 cup sharp cheddar cheese, shredded
- ¼ cup scallions, finely chopped

Preparation:

1. Preheat oven to 350° F. Grease a 9 x 13-inch baking dish.

2. In a large skillet, heat olive oil over medium-low heat.

3. Sauté cubed chicken until done. Drain any remaining liquid from skillet.

4. Toss chicken with chili powder, cumin, garlic powder, onion powder, salt and pepper. Transfer chicken to the prepared baking dish.

5. In a bowl, combine sour cream, chilies and salsa. Pour mixture over chicken.

6. Bake chicken for 20-25 minutes.

7. Remove chicken from oven and top with shredded Monterey and cheddar cheeses. Return to oven for additional 5 minutes, or until cheese is melted.

8. Allow to cool slightly, top with chopped scallions and serve.

Per serving:

Calories 434; Fat: 25g; Carbs: 7g; Protein: 44g.

Stuffed Bacon Cheeseburgers

This recipe yields 4 servings.

Ingredients:

- 1½ lb lean ground beef
- ½ teaspoon salt
- ½ teaspoon black pepper
- Pinch of cayenne pepper
- 1 cup sharp cheddar cheese, shredded
- 4 slices bacon, cooked and crumbled
- ¼ cup green onions, finely chopped

Preparation:

1. Preheat grill to medium-high heat.

2. In a large bowl, thoroughly combine ground beef, ½ cup cheese, salt, black pepper and cayenne pepper. Form 8 thin patties.

3. In a separate bowl, combine remaining cheese, crumbled bacon and green onions.

4. Divide cheese and bacon mixture evenly

between 4 patties. Sandwich remaining patties on top, sealing at the edges.

5. Grill burgers for about 5 minutes on each side. Serve.

Per serving:

Calories 658; Fat: 47g; Carbs: 0.5g; Protein: 56g.

Broccoli Beef Bake

This recipe yields 8 servings.

Ingredients:

- 1½ cups almond flour
- 1 cup flax meal
- 1 tablespoon coconut flour
- ½ teaspoon salt, plus 1 teaspoon
- 3 tablespoons butter, melted
- 3 eggs
- 1 lb lean ground beef
- 1 teaspoon pepper
- ½ teaspoon cumin
- 1 cup sharp cheddar cheese, shredded
- 1 cup Monterey Jack cheese, shredded
- ½ cup pepper jack cheese, shredded
- 1½ cups broccoli florets, finely chopped
- 3 tablespoons sour cream
- ½ teaspoon dried oregano
- ½ teaspoon dried basil

Preparation:

1. Preheat oven to 400° F. Grease 9-inch springform pan.

2. In a large bowl, combine almond flour, flax meal, coconut flour and ½ teaspoon of salt.

3. In a separate bowl, whisk together melted butter and 1 egg. Stir into flour mixture.

4. Spread dough evenly in prepared pan, covering the bottom and a little on the sides. Bake for 10 minutes.

5. While pie crust is baking, sauté beef in a large skillet until no longer pink. Drain fat, and season with 1 teaspoon salt, 1 teaspoon pepper and ½ teaspoon cumin.

6. Whisk 2 remaining eggs in a large bowl, and add shredded cheese, broccoli florets, sour cream, dried oregano and basil. Mix well.

7. Spread beef evenly on top of pie crust. Top with cheese mixture.

8. Return to oven for 15 minutes.

9. Remove from oven, and allow to cool for another 15 minutes. Release from pan, slice and serve.

Per serving:

Calories 692; Fat: 54g; Carbs: 12g; Protein: 41g.

Deep Dish Pizza

This recipe yields 4 servings.

Ingredients:

- 1 tablespoon cream cheese, softened
- 1 egg
- ¼ cup heavy cream
- 1 tablespoon Parmesan cheese, freshly grated
- ½ teaspoon dried oregano
- ½ teaspoon garlic powder
- 1 cup Monterey Jack cheese, shredded
- ½ cup marinara sauce
- 1 cup mozzarella cheese, shredded
- 8 slices bacon, cooked and crumbled

Preparation:

1. Preheat oven to 375° F. Grease 9-inch pie plate.

2. In a bowl, whisk together cream cheese and egg. Add heavy cream, Parmesan cheese,

dried oregano and garlic powder; combine well.

3. Spread Monterey Jack cheese onto bottom of pie plate. Top with egg mixture.

4. Bake crust for 15 minutes; remove from oven and cool for 5 minutes.

5. Coat crust with marinara sauce, mozzarella cheese and crumbled bacon.

6. Return to oven for another 15 minutes.

7. Let cool for 10 minutes, slice and serve.

Per serving:

Calories 475; Fat: 39g; Carbs: 4g; Protein: 27g.

Stuffed Cabbage Enchiladas

This recipe yields 4 servings.

Ingredients:

- 2 tablespoons butter
- 4 boneless, skinless chicken breasts
- 1 head white cabbage
- 1 cup chicken broth
- 1 cup sour cream
- 8 oz fire-roasted canned green chilies
- ¼ cup cilantro, chopped
- 1 cup pepper jack cheese, shredded
- 1 large avocado, sliced

Preparation:

1. Preheat oven to 350° F. Grease 8x8-inch baking dish.

2. In a large skillet, melt 2 tablespoons of butter over medium heat.

3. Season chicken breasts with salt and pepper, and sauté until cooked through.

4. While chicken is cooking, bring a large pot of water to a boil.

5. Carefully peel whole leaves off the head of cabbage and drop into boiling water. Allow to cook for 2-3 minutes, and then set onto a paper towel to dry.

6. In a separate pot, bring chicken broth to a boil over medium heat. Reduce heat to low, and add sour cream and chilies. Simmer sauce until thickened slightly and heated through, being careful not to let it boil.

7. Pour a thin layer of sauce into prepared baking dish.

8. Shred cooked chicken and mix with cilantro and ½ cup cheese. Spoon chicken into cabbage leaves, roll and place in baking dish. Cover stuffed cabbage with remaining sauce and cheese.

9. Bake for 25-30 minutes.

10. Serve with sliced avocado.

Per serving:

Calories 549; Fat: 34g; Carbs: 14g; Protein: 47g.

Hoisin-Soy Pork Tenderloin

This recipe yields 4 servings.

Ingredients:

- 1 lb pork tenderloin, cut into 3" strips
- 1 teaspoon salt
- 3 tablespoons hoisin sauce
- 2 tablespoons soy sauce
- 1 tablespoon vinegar
- 3 tablespoons peanut oil
- 1 garlic clove, minced
- 3 cups Napa cabbage, thinly sliced
- 1 red bell pepper; cored, seeded and thinly sliced

Preparation:

1. Season pork with salt.

2. In a small bowl, combine hoisin, soy sauce and balsamic vinegar.

3. In a large non-stick skillet, heat 2 tablespoons of peanut oil over medium-high

heat. Once the oil is heated, add pork and cook for about 2 minutes. Remove to plate.

4. Add remaining peanut oil to skillet and sauté garlic. Add cabbage and bell pepper, and cook for about 2 minutes. Season with salt and pepper.

5. Pour hoisin mixture into skillet with pork, and cook for about a minute.

6. Remove skillet from heat and let stand for 2 minutes. Serve.

Per serving:

Calories 340; Fat: 18g; Carbs: 9g; Protein: 34g.

SMOOTHIES

Ginger Grapefruit Green Smoothie

Serves 1 / Prep time: 10 minutes

Ingredients:

- ½ a peeled grapefruit
- 1 small chunk fresh ginger
- 1 cup fresh spinach
- 1 handful fresh parsley
- 1 cup water
- 1 cup ice

Preparation:

1. Place all of the ingredients except the ice into your blender and blend until smooth.

2. Add the ice and blend for another minute until the ice is crushed.

Per serving:

Calories: 48; Fat: 0g; Protein: 2g; Carbs: 11g; Fiber: 2g; Net Carbs: 9g.

Tropical Kiwi Smoothie

Serves 1 / Prep time: 5 minutes

Ingredients:

- 1 peeled kiwi
- 1 cup coconut water
- ½ an avocado
- 1 cup baby spinach
- 1 handful fresh mint leaves
- 1 cup ice

Preparation:

1. Place all of the ingredients except the ice into your blender and blend until smooth.

2. Add in the ice and blend for another minute until the ice is crushed

Per serving:

Calories: 4258; Fat: 20g; Protein: 4g; Carbs: 21g; Fiber: 10g; Net Carbs: 11g.

Veggie-Packed Green Smoothie

Serves 1 / Prep time: 5 minutes

Ingredients:

- 4 large kale leaves
- 3 celery stalks
- 1 medium cucumber
- 2 lemons (peeled)
- handful fresh parsley

Preparation:

Place all of the ingredients through a juicer, and enjoy right away.

Per serving:

Calories: 128; Fat: 1g; Protein: 6g; Carbs: 18g; Fiber: 8g; Net Carbs: 9g.

Cucumber Lemonade

Serves: 1 / Prep time 5 minutes

Ingredients:

- 2 cucumbers
- 4 celery stalks
- 2 lemons (peeled)

Preparation:

Run all of the ingredients through a juicer, and enjoy right away.

Per serving:

Calories: 108; Fat: 1g; Protein: 5g; Carbs: 19g; Fiber: 9g; Net Carbs: 8g.

Tropical Raspberry Smoothie

Serves 1 / Prep time: 5 minutes

Ingredients:

- 1 cup of frozen raspberries
- ¼ cup silken organic tofu
- ½ cup unsweetened coconut milk
- 1 teaspoon sugar-free sweetener
- 1 cup ice
- Fresh mint leaves (optional garnish)

Preparation:

1. Place all of the ingredients into the blender except for the ice and the stevia. Blend until smooth.
2. Add in the ice and stevia and blend for another minute.
3. Taste and if needed, adjust the sweetness by adding another pinch of stevia.
4. Garnish with fresh mint leaves and serve.

Per serving:

Calories: 381; Fat: 32g; Protein: 8g; Carbs: 21g; Fiber: 11g; Net Carbs: 10g.

Raspberry Almond Smoothie

Serves 1 / Prep time: 10 minutes

Ingredients:

- ½ cup frozen raspberries
- 2 tablespoons unsalted almonds
- ½ cup unsweetened almond milk
- 1 scoop vanilla protein powder
- Toasted almond slices (optional garnish)

Preparation:

1. Place all of the ingredients, except the optional garnish, into your blender and blend until smooth.
2. Additional almond milk may be needed to reach desired consistency.
3. Garnish with toasted almond slices, if desired, and serve.

Per serving:

Calories: 303; Fat: 12g; Protein: 26g; Carbs: 20g; Fiber: 9g; Net Carbs: 11g.

Gingered Plum Smoothie

Serves 2 / Prep time: 10 minutes

Ingredients:

- 1 cup frozen plum pieces
- ½ cup chopped raw beet
- 1 small piece fresh ginger (about ½ ")
- ½ cup canned coconut milk
- 1 cup water
- 1 tablespoon almond butter
- 1 tablespoon coconut oil
- ¼ teaspoon cinnamon
- ½ cup ice

Preparation:

1. Place all ingredients into your blender and blend until smooth and creamy.

2. Serve immediately or store in the fridge for later.
Per serving:

Calories: 281; Fat: 26g; Protein: 6g; Carbs:

11g; Fiber: 3g; Net Carbs: 8g.

Avocado Fat Burning Smoothie

Serves: 1 Prep time: 10 minutes

Ingredients:

- ½ of an avocado
- ½ kiwi fruit
- 1 tablespoon fresh lime juice
- 1 tablespoon chopped chives
- ½ cup unsweetened almond milk
- 1 tablespoon heavy cream
- ½ cup ice
- Pinch of sea salt

Preparation:

1. Place all of the ingredients except for the ice into your blender and blend until smooth.

2. Add the ice and blend until the ice is crushed.

3. Serve and enjoy!

Per serving:

Calories: 189; Fat: 17g; Protein: 2g; Carbs: 10g; Fiber: 5g; Net Carbs: 5g.

Nutty Fat Bomb Smoothie

Serves 2 / Time: 5 minute

Ingredients:

- 1 cup canned coconut milk
- 1 cup unsweetened almond milk
- 2 tablespoons coconut oil
- 2 tablespoons peanut butter
- 1 teaspoon sugar-free sweetener
- ½ teaspoon vanilla extract
- ½ teaspoon cinnamon
- 1 cup ice

Preparation:

1. Starting with the ice, add all ingredients into a blender.
2. Blend until smooth.
3. Can be enjoyed immediately or stored in the fridge for later use, though you may have to give a good stir to mix any ingredients that have settled.

Per serving:

Calories: 507; Fat: 52g; Protein: 7g; Carbs: 11g; Fiber: 4g; Net Carbs: 7g.

Cinnamon Roll Smoothie

Serves 2 / Prep time: 5 minutes

Ingredients:

- 2 cups unsweetened almond milk
- ½ cup plain yogurt
- 1 scoop vanilla protein powder
- 1 teaspoon cinnamon
- ½ teaspoon vanilla extract
- 1 teaspoon ground flax seeds
- 1 teaspoon sugar-free sweetener
- 1 cup ice

Preparation:

1. Place all of the ingredients except the ice into your blender and blend until smooth.
2. Add the ice and blend for another minute until the ice is crushed.
3. Garnish with a sprinkle of cinnamon and serve immediately.
Per serving:

Calories: 154; Fat: 6g; Protein: 16g; Carbs: 9g; Fiber: 2g; Net Carbs: 7g.

Minty Keto Milkshake

Serves 1 / Prep time: 10 minutes

Ingredients:

- 1 cup fresh spinach
- ½ teaspoon peppermint extract
- ½ an avocado
- 1 scoop vanilla protein powder
- 1 cup unsweetened almond milk
- 8-10 drops liquid stevia, to taste
- 1 cup ice

Preparation:

1. Place the avocado, spinach, protein powder, and milk in a blender and blend until smooth.
2. Add the liquid stevia, peppermint extract, and ice. Blend until smooth.
3. Taste and add additional stevia or peppermint, if desired.
4. Serve and enjoy!
Per serving:

Calories: 372; Fat: 25g; Protein: 26g; Carbs: 15g; Fiber: 8g; Net Carbs: 7g.

Pineapple Green Smoothie

Serves 1 / Prep time: 5 minutes

Ingredients:

- ¼ cup pineapple cubes
- 1 cucumber
- 2 celery stalks
- ½ a green apple
- 3 large romaine leaves
- 1 small nub fresh ginger, grated

Preparation:

Place all of the ingredients through a juicer, and chill for 30 minutes before serving.

Per serving:

Calories: 58; Fat: 1g; Protein: 2g; Carbs: 12g; Fiber: 4g; Net Carbs: 8g.

Chocolate Peanut Butter Shake

Serves 1 / Prep time: 5 minutes

Ingredients:

- 1 tablespoon cocoa powder
- 1 scoop chocolate protein powder
- 1 tablespoon peanut butter
- 1 cup unsweetened almond milk
- 1 cup ice

Preparation:

1. Place all of the ingredients except for the ice into your blender and blend until smooth.
2. Add in the ice, and blend for another minute until the ice is crushed.
3. Serve right away.

Per serving:

Calories: 266; Fat: 14g; Protein: 28g; Carbs: 12g; Fiber: 4g; Net Carbs: 8g.

Strawberry Cheesecake Smoothie

Serves 1 / Prep time: 5 minutes

Ingredients:

- ½ cup frozen strawberries
- ½ cup reduced-fat cottage cheese
- 1 cup unsweetened almond milk
- 1 teaspoon vanilla extract
- 1 teaspoon stevia
- 1 cup ice
- Optional Garnish
- Fresh strawberries

Preparation:

1. Place all of the ingredients except for the ice into your blender and blend until smooth.

2. Add the ice, and blend for another minute until the ice is crushed.

3. Garnish with fresh strawberry, if desired, and serve immediately.

Per serving:

Calories: 161; Fat: 5g; Protein: 16g; Carbs: 12g; Fiber: 3g; Net Carbs: 9g.

USEFUL TIPS AND TRICKS

Ketogenic diet tips are described here to run off from the ketone bodies and fatty acids that are most of the time useless in the human body. This ketogenic diet plan not only reduces the chances of the chronic disease, but also helps in fat metabolism and development of the muscles in the body. In the cyclic ketogenic diet, the person or patient will go for low carbohydrates for three days and after that one can have a bit higher carbohydrate. The method of stay hydrated is considered as the no-brainer, although this method is not so easy for the person who wants to follow it, but anyone can follow this if he or she wants to stay hydrated.

The main reason behind this idea that this method is difficult to follow is that people often stay busy in their daily routine life and they don't get time to follow this method. In this method the person who wants to be hydrated needs to drink the water of 32 oz daily, he or she can also have tea or coffee instead of water within an hour of waking up in the morning. After drinking that 32 oz of water or other drink he or she should drink some 32 to 48 oz of juice water or any other drink except alcohol in the afternoon.

In this method, the person should follow these instructions of experts:

- Eat light and use tea or coffee in the morning time.
- Eating light makes the digestive system to digest the food easily.
- Do not drink water after eating food.
- Avoid eating if you are not hungry enough.
- Must follow the given diet for a long time.

The reason behind this method of the ketogenic diet is that the high amount of water after eating food is not beneficial for the health of the person, because the stomach of the person fails to digest the food easily. So this is harmful to the person's digestive system and I always say that the person, whether there is a male or a female, should drink water or any other drink before eating food and avoid drinking water after eating food.

According to my knowledge, the person, whether there is a male or female, he or she should drink water half of the weight of his or her body in ounces of water. If he or she can drink water closer or equal to the full body weight of his or her own, then he or she should drink this much water. For example, if the person has a body weight of 160 lbs, then he or she should drink 140 to 160 ounce of water, and even if he or she can drink 180 ounces of water, then this is also good for his or her health. But the person should mind the timing of drinking water, as I said before, he or she should drink before eating food or at least 3 hours after eating food. Some of the important points of the ketogenic diet are in the lines below:

- A person should drink water in ounces equal or half of his or her body weight.
- Try intermittent fasting at least for 20 to 30 days.
- Do not drink or eat during the practice of intermittent fasting period.
- Avoid heavy meals right after the intermittent fasting period.
- Continues practice is mandatory for the good results of intermittent fasting.

Once the person starts following this method of eating and drinking, he or she will find this easy and will continue it for a long time. Another way of the ketogenic diet is intermittent fasting. This way of ketogenic diet is very beneficial for all of the people except those who are suffering from diseases. The reason behind this argument is that intermittent fasting always reduce calories from the body, and the body do not consume carbs or protein, this is the best way of going low carb. The person, who wants to practice intermittent fasting, should practice it at least for twenty to thirty days and he or she will find that this is the best method of the ketogenic diet.

AUTHOR'S NOTE

Before starting a ketogenic diet plan, one should consult with a medical practitioner. This is mandatory for you to be informed of any pre-existing health conditions.

Thanks again for downloading and reading this book, I hope you enjoy it! Please consider leaving a review. Readers rely on reviews, as do authors.

www.ingramcontent.com/pod-product-compliance
Lightning Source LLC
Chambersburg PA
CBHW020513290526
45786CB00002B/587